The Ultimate Guide To Juicing for Weight Loss

Sip Your Way to a Slimmer, Healthier You

Melissa Fogel

Table Of Contents

Introduction

Conclusion

Introduction

Juicing has become a popular trend in recent years, especially for those looking to lose weight. It involves extracting the juice from fruits and vegetables, which is packed with nutrients, vitamins, and minerals that can help promote weight loss and improve overall health.

Juicing for weight loss is not a quick fix solution, but rather a sustainable lifestyle change that can lead to long-term weight management. It can be a great way to incorporate more fruits and vegetables into your diet, which are essential for maintaining a healthy weight.

In this guide, we will explore the benefits of juicing for weight loss, the science behind it, how to choose the right juicer for your needs, essential ingredients for weight loss juices, top recipes to try, tips for incorporating juicing into your daily routine, common mistakes to avoid, how to prepare for a successful juicing cleanse, and frequently asked questions about juicing for weight loss.

By the end of this guide, you will have a better understanding of how juicing can help you achieve your weight loss goals and how to make it a sustainable part of your lifestyle.

Chapter 1: Understanding the benefits of juicing

Juicing for weight loss is not a quick fix solution, but rather a sustainable lifestyle change that can lead to long-term weight management. It can be a great way to incorporate more fruits and vegetables into your diet, which are essential for maintaining The Science Behind Juicing for Weight Loss

Juicing for weight loss is not just a fad or trend – there is actual science behind it. Here are some of the ways that juicing can help you lose weight:

1. **Boosts metabolism:** Certain ingredients in weight loss juices, such as ginger and cayenne pepper, can

help boost your metabolism, which in turn helps you burn more calories throughout the day.

2. **Reduces inflammation:** Chronic inflammation in the body can lead to weight gain and other health issues. Many fruits and vegetables used in juicing, such as leafy greens and berries, are high in antioxidants that can help reduce inflammation.

3. **Promotes satiety:** Juicing can help you feel fuller for longer, which can prevent overeating and snacking on unhealthy foods. This is because the fiber in fruits and vegetables slows down digestion and keeps you feeling satisfied.

4. **Provides essential nutrients:** Juicing is a great way to get a variety of essential nutrients, such as

vitamins and minerals, that your body needs to function properly. When your body is getting all the nutrients it needs, it can function more efficiently and burn calories more effectively.

5. Cleanses the body: Juicing can help cleanse your body of toxins and waste that may be contributing to weight gain. This is especially true if you incorporate ingredients like lemon or dandelion greens, which are natural diuretics that help flush out excess fluids.

Chapter 2: The science behind juicing for weight loss

1. Nutrient Density

One of the main benefits of juicing is that it allows you to consume a large amount of nutrients in a small volume of liquid. Vitamins, minerals, and antioxidants that are crucial for optimum health are abundant in fruits and vegetables. By juicing them, you can extract all of these nutrients and consume them in an easily digestible form.

2. Fiber Content

While juicing can be a great way to increase your nutrient intake, it does have one major drawback: it removes the fiber from fruits and vegetables. In addition to being beneficial for your digestive system, fiber can make you feel content and full after meals. Without it, you may be more likely to overeat or snack on unhealthy foods.

3. Caloric Intake
Another factor to consider when juicing for weight loss is the number of calories you are consuming. While fruits and vegetables are generally low in calories, some juices can still be quite high in sugar and calories. It's important to choose ingredients carefully and monitor your overall caloric intake to ensure that you are not consuming more calories than you are burning.

4. Meal Replacement
Some people use juicing as a meal replacement strategy for weight loss. While this can be effective in the short term, it's important to ensure

that you are still getting all of the nutrients and calories your body needs to function properly. Juicing should not be used as a long-term solution for weight loss.

5. Exercise
Finally, it's important to remember that juicing alone is not enough to achieve significant weight loss. Exercise is also an essential component of any weight loss plan. By combining juicing with regular exercise, you can create a healthy and sustainable lifestyle that will help you achieve your weight loss goals.

Chapter 3: Essential ingredients for weight loss juices

Juicing can be a great way to support weight loss goals, as long as you choose the right ingredients. Here are some essential ingredients to include in your weight loss juices:

1. Leafy Greens: Leafy greens such as kale, spinach, and collard greens are packed with nutrients and fiber, which can help keep you full and satisfied. They are also low in calories, making them a great addition to weight loss juices.

2. Citrus Fruits: Citrus fruits such as oranges, lemons, and grapefruits are high in vitamin C and antioxidants, which can help support a healthy

immune system and promote weight loss. They also add a refreshing flavor to juices.

3. Berries: Berries such as blueberries, raspberries, and strawberries are low in calories and high in fiber and antioxidants. They can help regulate blood sugar levels and promote satiety, making them a great addition to weight loss juices.

4. Ginger: Ginger has been shown to have anti-inflammatory and metabolism-boosting properties, making it a great addition to weight loss juices. It also adds a spicy kick to juices.

5. Cucumber: Cucumbers are low in calories and high in water content, making them a great addition to weight loss juices. They also add a

refreshing flavor and can help flush out toxins from the body.

6. Apple: Apples are high in fiber and antioxidants, which can help regulate blood sugar levels and promote satiety. They also add a sweet flavor to juices.

7. Carrots: Carrots are high in beta-carotene and fiber, which can help support a healthy immune system and promote weight loss. They also add a sweet flavor to juices.

Chapter 4: Recipes for weight loss juices

1. Green Detox Juice

Ingredients:
- 1 cucumber
- 2 celery stalks
- 1 green apple
- 1 lemon
- 1 inch ginger root
- Handful of spinach

Instructions:
1. Wash all ingredients.
2. Cut the cucumber, celery, and apple into small pieces.
3. Peel the lemon and ginger.
4. Add all ingredients to a juicer and juice.
5. Serve and enjoy!

2. Carrot and Orange Juice

Ingredients:
- 4 large carrots
- 2 oranges

Instructions:
1. Wash all ingredients.
2. Peel the oranges and cut them into small pieces.
3. Cut the carrots into small pieces.
4. Add all ingredients to a juicer and juice.
5. Serve and enjoy!

3. Beet and Berry Juice

Ingredients:
- 2 beets
- 1 cup mixed berries (strawberries, blueberries, raspberries)
- 1 orange

Instructions:
1. Wash all ingredients.
2. Cut the beets into small pieces.
3. Peel the orange and cut it into small pieces.
4. Add all ingredients to a juicer and juice.
5. Serve and enjoy!

4. Pineapple and Kale Juice

Ingredients:
- 1/2 pineapple
- 2 cups kale
- 1 lemon

Instructions:
1. Wash all ingredients.
2. Cut the pineapple into small pieces.
3. Cut the kale into small pieces.
4. Peel the lemon.
5. Add all ingredients to a juicer and juice. Serve and enjoy

5. Cucumber and Mint Juice

Ingredients:

- 2 cucumbers
- Handful of mint leaves
- 1 lime

Instructions:

1. Wash all ingredients.
2. Cut the cucumbers into small pieces.
3. Remove the mint leaves from the stems.
4. Peel the lime.
5. Add all ingredients to a juicer and juice.
6. Serve and enjoy!

6. Spinach and Apple Juice

Ingredients:

- 2 cups spinach
- 2 green apples
- 1 lemon

Instructions:
1. Wash all ingredients.
2. Cut the apples into small pieces.
3. Remove the stems from the spinach.
4. Peel the lemon.
5. Add all ingredients to a juicer and juice.
6. Serve and enjoy!

7. Watermelon and Mint Juice

Ingredients:
- 1/2 watermelon
- Handful of mint leaves
- 1 lime

Instructions:
1. Wash all ingredients.
2. Cut the watermelon into small pieces.
3. Remove the mint leaves from the stems.
4. Peel the lime.

5. Add all ingredients to a juicer and juice.
6. Serve and enjoy!

8. Carrot and Ginger Juice

Ingredients:
- 4 large carrots
- 1 inch ginger root
- 1 orange

Instructions:
1. Wash all ingredients.
2. Cut the carrots into small pieces.
3. Peel the ginger and cut it into small pieces.
4. Peel the orange and cut it into small pieces.
5. Add all ingredients to a juicer and juice.
6. Serve and enjoy!

9. Blueberry and Kale Juice

Ingredients:
- 1 cup blueberries
- 2 cups kale
- 1 lemon

Instructions:
1. Wash all ingredients.
2. Cut the kale into small pieces.
3. Peel the lemon.
4. Add all ingredients to a juicer and juice.
5. Serve and enjoy!

10. Beet and Carrot Juice

Ingredients:
- 2 beets
- 4 large carrots
- Handful of parsley

Instructions:
1. Wash all ingredients.
2. Cut the beets and carrots into small pieces.
3. Remove the stems from the parsley.
4. Add all ingredients to a juicer and juice.
5. Serve and enjoy!

11. Pineapple and Ginger Juice
Ingredients:
- 1/2 pineapple
- 1 inch ginger root
- Handful of cilantro

Instructions:
1. Wash all ingredients.
2. Cut the pineapple into small pieces.
3. Peel the ginger and cut it into small pieces.

4. Remove the stems from the cilantro.

5. Add all ingredients to a juicer and juice. After that, serve and enjoy.

12. Orange and Carrot Juice

Ingredients:

- 4 large carrots

- 2 oranges

Instructions:

1. Wash all ingredients.

2. Peel the oranges and cut them into small pieces.

3. Cut the carrots into small pieces.

4. Add all ingredients to a juicer and juice. Serve and enjoy.

13. Apple and Cucumber Juice

Ingredients:

- 2 green apples

- 2 cucumbers

- Handful of parsley

Instructions:
1. Wash all ingredients.
2. Cut the apples and cucumbers into small pieces.
3. Remove the stems from the parsley.
4. Add all ingredients to a juicer and juice.
5. Serve and enjoy!

14. Watermelon and Lime Juice

Ingredients:
- 1/2 watermelon
- 2 limes

Instructions:
1. Wash all ingredients.
2. Cut the watermelon into small pieces.
3. Peel the limes and cut them into small pieces.

4. Add all ingredients to a juicer and juice.
5. Serve and enjoy

15. Spinach and Pineapple Juice
Ingredients:
- 2 cups spinach
- 1/2 pineapple
- 1 lemon

Instructions:
1. Wash all ingredients.
2. Cut the pineapple into small pieces.
3. Remove the stems from the spinach.
4. Peel the lemon.
5. Add all ingredients to a juicer and juice.
6. Serve and enjoy!

16. Carrot and Beet Juice

Ingredients:
- 4 large carrots
- 2 beets
- Handful of parsley

Instructions:
1. Wash all ingredients.
2. Cut the carrots and beets into small pieces.
3. Remove the stems from the parsley.
4. Add all ingredients to a juicer and juice.
5. Serve and enjoy!

17. Blueberry and Cucumber Juice

Ingredients:
- 1 cup blueberries
- 2 cucumbers
- Handful of mint leaves

Instructions:

1. Wash all ingredients.

2. Cut the cucumbers into small pieces.

3. Remove the mint leaves from the stems.

4. Add all ingredients to a juicer and juice.

5. Serve and enjoy!

18. Pineapple and Mint Juice

Ingredients:

- 1/2 pineapple

- Handful of mint leaves

- 1 lime

Instructions:

1. Wash all ingredients.

2. Cut the pineapple into small pieces.

3. Remove the mint leaves from the stems.

4. Peel the lime.

5. Add all ingredients to a juicer and juice.
6. Serve and enjoy!

19. Carrot and Orange Juice with Turmeric

Ingredients:
- 4 large carrots
- 2 oranges
- 1 inch turmeric root

Instructions:
1. Wash all ingredients.
2. Peel the oranges and cut them into small pieces.
3. Cut the carrots into small pieces.
4. Peel the turmeric root and cut it into small pieces.
5. Add all ingredients to a juicer and juice.
6. Serve and enjoy!

20. Green Apple and Cucumber Juice

Ingredients:
- 2 green apples
- 2 cucumbers
- Handful of kale

Instructions:
1. Wash all ingredients.
2. Cut the apples and cucumbers into small pieces.
3. Remove the stems from the kale.
4. Add all ingredients to a juicer and juice.
5. Serve and enjoy!

21. Carrot and Pineapple Juice

Ingredients:
- 4 large carrots
- 1/2 pineapple
- Handful of mint leaves

Instructions:

1. Wash all ingredients.

2. Cut the carrots and pineapple into small pieces.

3. Remove the mint leaves from the stems.

4. Add all ingredients to a juicer and juice.

5. Serve and enjoy!

22. Green Detox Juice with Turmeric

Ingredients:

- 1 cucumber
- 2 celery stalks
- 1 green apple
- 1 lemon
- 1 inch ginger root
- Handful of spinach
- 1 inch turmeric root

Instructions:
1. Wash all ingredients.
2. Cut the cucumber, celery, and apple into small pieces.
3. Peel the lemon, ginger, and turmeric root.
4. Add all ingredients to a juicer and juice.
5. Serve and enjoy!

23. Beet and Orange Juice

Ingredients:
- 2 beets
- 2 oranges
- Handful of cilantro

Instructions:
1. Wash all ingredients.
2. Cut the beets and oranges into small pieces.

3. Remove the stems from the cilantro.

4. Add all ingredients to a juicer and juice.

5. Serve and enjoy!

24. Pineapple and Cucumber Juice

Ingredients:
- 1/2 pineapple
- 2 cucumbers
- Handful of parsley

Instructions:

1. Wash all ingredients.

2. Cut the pineapple and cucumbers into small pieces.

3. Remove the stems from the parsley.

4. Add all ingredients to a juicer and juice.

5. Serve and enjoy!

25. Carrot and Spinach Juice

Ingredients:

- 4 large carrots
- 2 cups spinach
- 1 lemon

Instructions:

1. Wash all ingredients.
2. Cut the carrots into small pieces.
3. Remove the stems from the spinach.
4. Peel the lemon.
5. Add all ingredients to a juicer and juice.
6. Serve and enjoy!

26. Blueberry and Pineapple Juice

Ingredients:

- 1 cup blueberries
- 1/2 pineapple
- Handful of mint leaves

Instructions:

1. Wash all ingredients.

2. Cut the pineapple into small pieces.

3. Remove the mint leaves from the stems.

4. Add all ingredients to a juicer and juice.

5. Serve and enjoy!

27. Watermelon and Cucumber Juice

Ingredients:

- 1/2 watermelon
- 2 cucumbers
- Handful of basil leaves

Instructions:

1. Wash all ingredients.

2. Cut the watermelon and cucumbers into small pieces.

3. Remove the stems from the basil leaves.

4. Add all ingredients to a juicer and juice.

5. Serve and enjoy!

28. Carrot and Kale Juice

Ingredients:

- 4 large carrots
- 2 cups kale
- 1 lemon

Instructions:

1. Wash all ingredients.
2. Cut the carrots into small pieces.
3. Remove the stems from the kale.
4. Peel the lemon.
5. Add all ingredients to a juicer and juice.
6. Serve and enjoy!

29. Pineapple and Orange Juice

Ingredients:
- 1/2 pineapple
- 2 oranges
- Handful of mint leaves

Instructions:
1. Wash all ingredients.
2. Cut the pineapple into small pieces.
3. Peel the oranges and cut them into small pieces.
4. Remove the mint leaves from the stems.
5. Add all ingredients to a juicer and juice.
6. Serve and enjoy!

30. Beet and Kale Juice

Ingredients:
- 2 beets
- 2 cups kale
- 1 lemon

Instructions:
1. Wash all ingredients.
2. Cut the beets into small pieces.
3. Remove the stems from the kale.
4. Peel the lemon.
5. Add all ingredients to a juicer and juice.
6. Serve and enjoy!

31. Watermelon and Mint Juice with Turmeric

Ingredients:
- 1/2 watermelon
- Handful of mint leaves
- 1 inch turmeric root

Instructions:
1. Wash all ingredients.
2. Cut the watermelon into small pieces.
3. Remove the mint leaves from the stems.

4. Peel the turmeric root and cut it into small pieces.
5. Add all ingredients to a juicer and juice.
6. Serve and enjoy!

32. Blueberry and Orange Juice
Ingredients:
- 1 cup blueberries
- 2 oranges
- Handful of basil leaves

Instructions:
1. Wash all ingredients.
2. Peel the oranges and cut them into small pieces.
3. Remove the stems from the basil leaves.
4. Add all ingredients to a juicer and juice.
5. Serve and enjoy!

33. Pineapple and Ginger Juice with Turmeric

Ingredients:
- 1/2 pineapple
- 1 inch ginger root
- Handful of cilantro
- 1 inch turmeric root

Instructions:
1. Wash all ingredients.
2. Cut the pineapple into small pieces.
3. Peel the ginger, cilantro, and turmeric root.
4. Add all ingredients to a juicer and juice.
5. Serve and enjoy!

34. Carrot and Watermelon Juice

Ingredients:
- 4 large carrots
- 1/2 watermelon

- Handful of basil leaves

Instructions:
1. Wash all ingredients.
2. Cut the carrots and watermelon into small pieces.
3. Remove the stems from the basil leaves.
4. Add all ingredients to a juicer and juice.
5. Serve and enjoy!

35. Cucumber and Pineapple Juice

Ingredients:
- 2 cucumbers
- 1/2 pineapple
- Handful of mint leaves

Instructions:
1. Wash all ingredients.

2. Cut the cucumbers and pineapple into small pieces.
3. Remove the mint leaves from the stems.
4. Add all ingredients to a juicer and juice.
5. Serve and enjoy!

36. Beet and Pineapple Juice
Ingredients:
- 2 beets
- 1/2 pineapple
- Handful of cilantro

Instructions:
1. Wash all ingredients.
2. Cut the beets and pineapple into small pieces.
3. Remove the stems from the cilantro.
4. Add all ingredients to a juicer and juice. Serve and enjoy

37. Green Apple and Kale Juice

Ingredients:

- 2 green apples
- 2 cups kale
- 1 lemon

Instructions:

1. Wash all ingredients.
2. Cut the apples into small pieces.
3. Remove the stems from the kale.
4. Peel the lemon.
5. Add all ingredients to a juicer and juice.
6. Serve and enjoy!

38. Carrot and Blueberry Juice

Ingredients:

- 4 large carrots
- 1 cup blueberries
- Handful of parsley

Instructions:

1. Wash all ingredients.

2. Cut the carrots into small pieces.

3. Remove any stems from the blueberries.

4. Remove the stems from the parsley.

5. Add all ingredients to a juicer and juice.

6. Serve and enjoy!

39. Watermelon and Basil Juice

Ingredients:

- 1/2 watermelon
- Handful of basil leaves
- 1 lime

Instructions:

1. Wash all ingredients.

2. Cut the watermelon into small pieces.

3. Remove the basil leaves from the stems.

4. Peel the lime.
5. Add all ingredients to a juicer and juice.
6. Serve and enjoy!

40. Pineapple and Blueberry Juice

Ingredients:
- 1/2 pineapple
- 1 cup blueberries
- Handful of mint leaves

Instructions:
1. Wash all ingredients.
2. Cut the pineapple into small pieces.
3. Remove any stems from the blueberries.
4. Remove the mint leaves from the stems.
5. Add all ingredients to a juicer and juice.
6. Serve and enjoy!

41. Carrot and Watermelon Juice with Turmeric

Ingredients:
- 4 large carrots
- 1/2 watermelon
- 1 inch turmeric root

Instructions:
1. Wash all ingredients.
2. Cut the carrots and watermelon into small pieces.
3. Peel the turmeric root and cut it into small pieces.
4. Add all ingredients to a juicer and juice.
5. Serve and enjoy!

42. Beet and Mint Juice

Ingredients:
- 2 beets
- Handful of mint leaves
- 1 lemon

Instructions:
1. Wash all ingredients.
2. Cut the beets into small pieces.
3. Remove the mint leaves from the stems.
4. Peel the lemon.
5. Add all ingredients to a juicer and juice.
6. Serve and enjoy!

43. Pineapple and Cilantro Juice

Ingredients:
- 1/2 pineapple
- Handful of cilantro
- 1 lime

Instructions:
1. Wash all ingredients.
2. Cut the pineapple into small pieces.
3. Remove the cilantro leaves from the stems.

4. Peel the lime.
5. Add all ingredients to a juicer and juice.
6. Serve and enjoy!

44. Carrot and Pineapple Juice with Turmeric

Ingredients:
- 4 large carrots
- 1/2 pineapple
- 1 inch turmeric root

Instructions:
1. Wash all ingredients.
2. Cut the carrots and pineapple into small pieces.
3. Peel the turmeric root and cut it into small pieces.
4. Add all ingredients to a juicer and juice.
5. Serve and enjoy!

45. Blueberry and Watermelon Juice

Ingredients:
- 1 cup blueberries
- 1/2 watermelon
- Handful of basil leaves

Instructions:
1. Wash all ingredients.
2. Cut the watermelon into small pieces
3. Remove any stems from the blueberries.
4. Remove the basil leaves from the stems.
5. Add all ingredients to a juicer and juice.
6. Serve and enjoy!

Chapter 5: Tips for incorporating juicing into your daily routine

1. Start with a small amount: If you're new to juicing, start with a small amount of juice and gradually increase the amount as your body adjusts.

2. Choose fresh and organic produce: Use fresh and organic produce to ensure that you're getting the most nutrients from your juice.

3. Experiment with different combinations: Mix and match different fruits and vegetables to find the combinations that you enjoy the most.

4. Drink juice in the morning: Drinking juice in the morning can help kickstart your day and give you a boost of energy.

5. Use a high-quality juicer: Invest in a high-quality juicer that can extract the maximum amount of juice from your produce.

6. Drink juice on an empty stomach: Drinking juice on an empty stomach allows your body to absorb the nutrients more efficiently.

7. Incorporate juice into meals: Use juice as a base for smoothies or as a dressing for salads to incorporate it into your meals.

Chapter 6: Common mistakes to avoid when juicing for weight loss

a. Using too much fruit: While fruit is a healthy addition to your diet, it's also high in sugar. Using too much fruit in your juice can lead to a spike in blood sugar and cause you to feel hungry soon after drinking it. Stick to mostly vegetables with a little bit of fruit for sweetness.

b. Not including enough protein or fiber: Juicing can be low in protein and fiber, which are important for keeping you feeling full and satisfied. Consider adding protein powder or a handful of nuts to your juice, or drinking it alongside a high-fiber snack like a piece of fruit or some raw veggies.

c. Drinking too much juice: While juice can be a healthy addition to your diet, it shouldn't replace whole foods entirely. Drinking too much juice can lead to nutrient imbalances and leave you feeling unsatisfied. Aim to include juice as part of a balanced diet that includes plenty of whole foods.

d. Not drinking enough water: Juicing can be dehydrating, so it's important to drink plenty of water throughout the day to stay hydrated.

e. Not consulting with a healthcare professional: If you're using juicing as part of a weight loss plan, it's important to talk to your healthcare professional first. They can help you determine the best approach for your individual needs and make sure you're getting all the nutrients you need.

Chapter 7: Preparing for a successful juicing cleanse

Juicing cleanses have become increasingly popular as a way to detoxify the body and jumpstart weight loss. However, preparing for a successful juicing cleanse requires some planning and preparation. Here are a some tips to help you get started:

a. Set realistic goals: Before starting a juicing cleanse, it's important to set realistic goals for yourself. Determine how long you want to do the cleanse for and what your desired outcome is. Keep in mind that a juicing cleanse should not be used as a long-term weight loss solution.

b. Stock up on fresh produce: Juicing cleanses require a lot of fresh produce, so it's important to stock up on fruits and vegetables before starting the cleanse. Choose a variety of colorful produce to ensure that you're getting a wide range of nutrients.

c. Invest in a quality juicer: A good quality juicer is essential for a successful juicing cleanse. Look for a juicer that is easy to use and clean, and that can handle a variety of produce.

d. Prepare your body: Before starting a juicing cleanse, it's important to prepare your body by gradually reducing your intake of processed foods, caffeine, and alcohol. This will help minimize any withdrawal symptoms you may experience during the cleanse.

e. Plan your meals: While on a juicing cleanse, it's important to have a plan for your meals. Decide which juices you'll be drinking each day and when you'll be drinking them. You may also want to include some raw fruits and vegetables as snacks.

f. Stay hydrated: Juicing cleanses can be dehydrating, so it's important to drink plenty of water throughout the day to stay hydrated.

g. Take it easy: During a juicing cleanse, it's important to listen to your body and take it easy. Avoid strenuous exercise and give yourself plenty of rest and relaxation time.

Conclusion:

incorporating juicing into your weight loss journey can be a game-changer. Not only does it provide you with a delicious and nutritious way to consume your daily dose of fruits and vegetables, but it also helps you shed those extra pounds. By following the tips and recipes in this book, you can create a sustainable juicing routine that fits your lifestyle and goals. Remember to listen to your body, stay hydrated, and enjoy the process. With dedication and consistency, you can achieve your desired weight and improve your overall health. Here's to a happy and healthy juicing journey!

www.ingramcontent.com/pod-product-compliance
Lightning Source LLC
Chambersburg PA
CBHW071112260726
48661CB00006B/2581